WRITING
AS A
TREATMENT FOR CANCER

O O O O O O O

PROMPTS FOR HEALING YOUR LIFE
DURING THE CANCER JOURNEY

WRITING
AS A
TREATMENT FOR CANCER

○ ○ ○ ○ ○ ○ ○

PROMPTS FOR HEALING YOUR LIFE
DURING THE CANCER JOURNEY

HEIDI BRIGHT, MDIV

SUNSTONE
PRESS
SANTA FE

Sunstone books may be purchased for educational, business, or sales promotional use.
For information please write: Special Markets Department, Sunstone Press,
P.O. Box 2321, Santa Fe, New Mexico 87504-2321.
Printed on acid-free paper
⊗
eBook: 978-1-61139-533-4

Library of Congress Cataloging-in-Publication Data

Names: Bright, Heidi, 1961- author
Title: Writing as a treatment for cancer : prompts for healing your life
     during the cancer journey / Heidi Bright, MDiv.
Description: Santa Fe : Sunstone Press, [2025] | Summary: "Take a deep
     internal dive through hundreds of expressive writing prompts that can
     help you heal your life and survive beyond cancer"-- Provided by
     publisher.
Identifiers: LCCN 2025033396 | ISBN 9781632937599 paperback | ISBN
     9781632937605 hardcover | ISBN 9781611395334 epub
Subjects: LCSH: Cancer--Treatment | Cancer--Patients |
     Cancer--Psychological aspects | LCGFT: Writing prompts
Classification: LCC RC263 .B665 2025 | DDC 616.99406--dc23/eng/20250730

LC record available at https://lccn.loc.gov/2025033396

WWW.SUNSTONEPRESS.COM
SUNSTONE PRESS / POST OFFICE BOX 2321 / SANTA FE, NM 87504-2321 /USA
(505) 988-4418

О

CONTENTS

INTRODUCTION

In March 2009, my family doctor ordered an ultrasound for a hard mass in my lower abdomen. The diagnosis: benign uterine fibroids. I was told the chances of there being cancer were one in 10,000. Because I was so healthy, I saw no need to continue with invasive testing; I chose to work with the fibroid through nutritional supplements and tai chi exercises until I reached menopause, a time when such fibroids generally disappear.

But the fibroids grew and grew. By July I lay under the surgeon's knife. Out came my cancer-filled cervix, uterus, fallopian tubes, ovaries, and six inches of small intestine. Scans exposed a cancerous spot on my lung. The high-grade endometrial stromal sarcoma had metastasized, and I was flung headlong into the fight of—and for—my life.

My heroine's journey to survive stage IV of an incredibly rare and highly aggressive cancer took me deep into my soul and far away to specialized physicians. I chose to use both conventional methods and complementary healing treatments—a choice that most likely saved my life. A village of lovely people supported and prayed for me every step of the way.

One of the specialists I met early on was an integrative physician at The University of Texas MD Anderson Cancer Center, Michael Fisch, MD, who told me that writing just one time about my emotions could have a far-reaching impact on my survival. Because I already was a writer—albeit a professional with training as a journalist—I decided to give it a try.

Another way I sought emotional healing was through weekly sessions with a clinical psychologist. She taught me the value of feeling my emotions as sensations in my body without thinking about them. As it turns out, I believe this was a key component of my surviving the deadly diagnosis. When I added intensely emotional expressions to my frequent writing practice, I helped my body respond in healthy ways.

When we write about our feelings—not simply journaling about facts or events—we give ourselves space for positive outcomes. Scientific studies demonstrate the power of both feeling our difficult emotions and then expressing them through handwriting. By using pens to put their innermost thoughts and feelings on paper, people have been rewarded with a range of physical, emotional, and social benefits. For example, breast cancer patients in one study had fewer unscheduled doctor visits and fewer reported symptoms.[1] In a similar study involving kidney cancer patients, those who did expressive writing exercises also had fewer symptoms and enjoyed improved physical function.[2]

Writing down our emotions and our experiences can help us because it reconnects us with a felt sense of participating in our lives rather than being victims of circumstances.

As we write, our experiences and feelings become more real, yet also more manageable. We start to see the golden threads that have moved through our lives. We begin to stitch together a tapestry of events, creating a big picture that offers insights. When we weave together our feelings with our stories, we put ourselves back together and give our lives meaning. This can provide more clarity, improve our sense of connectedness, and strengthen our spiritual lives. All of this helps our bodies to mend.

How to Approach this Book

Writing by hand can be a challenge while undergoing conventional cancer treatment. As my chemotherapy treatments progressed, I found it increasingly difficult to hold a pen, much less write more than a few sentences at a time. Some options to discuss with your doctors for managing peripheral neuropathy include taking vitamin B6 with a vitamin

B complex; the supplement r-lipoic acid; and glutamine powder. If you start these nutrients ahead of time, it might prevent some nerve damage.

You may wish to have a pen that you find enjoyable to write with, so you feel a little more motivated to delve into your life. Alternatively, typing on the computer can provide many of the same benefits as writing by hand.

As you write, I would suggest the following:

You can approach this book in a variety of ways. You can take each question in sequence, skip ahead, or open to a random page and point without looking and answer the prompt where your finger lands. Approaching the prompts with curiosity will enhance what you gain.

Many sections start with hard questions. This is to assist you with moving from actual emotions, which can be difficult to feel and can be uncomfortable, into higher textures of love, joy, and peace. Patience will be an important companion as you write. If you stick with the process, you might uncover clues that will naturally move you in a happier direction, and then the more positive prompts will add richness.

If you find yourself getting really upset with a prompt or while writing, then stop. Walk away from the writing and wait until you feel more calm. Then consider selecting a less difficult question to write about.

Write when you are alone and won't be interrupted. Turn off all electronic devices, including background music, unless you are writing on a device.

While some prompts might seem like a waste of time, please understand that making a response might reveal some unexpected insight. It might lift you out of your normal thinking processes and provide a new perspective or bring about a positive change in your life. Simply be open. If it doesn't yield anything today, try again in a week or a month.

Writing moves our thoughts out of our heads and onto something external. This opens up a little bit of space within us and can relieve internal pressure.

As you write, ignore grammar, punctuation, and structure. This process is not about perfection, nor is it about making logical sense. Don't think. Don't judge. Just write. This is about getting the brain out of the control seat so you can gain deeper insights.

Write whatever comes up for you. Don't censor it. This will reflect your raw feelings and thoughts, which can be an important component of your finding inner healing. These feelings will be uncomfortable. However, if you allow them to be what they are and to pass through you, without attaching meaning to them, they will not hurt you. If you think about them, fight them, or act on them, they can get stuck and raise your level of discomfort throughout your day.

As you reflect and write, try to give some attention to what is happening within your body. Note where there is tension (are you gripping your pen more tightly than normal?), a temperature change (is your head feeling warmer?) or a different sensation (are butterflies bumping your belly?). You can record these as well to enhance your understanding of what is happening inside you.

As we form sentences, we have to be more logical in our way of thinking. The effort helps clarify what is going on inside our heads, so our thoughts become more coherent. Take advantage of this by trying to make as much sense out of your story as possible.

Some of what you write you will want to dispose of immediately. When I do these types of writing, I use scrap paper. I suggest having a plan for immediately shredding what you write. This will help you be more honest and authentic because you won't be afraid of someone else finding it. I usually take the pearls I gain and rewrite them in my journal as things I learned without including names of other people.

Keep your journal in a safe place where only you can access it. This allows for maximum privacy, freedom, and authenticity.

Because a cancer diagnosis usually leaves us feeling completely out of control, use the prompts to guide you toward creating fresh options in your life. This will give you a sense for having some life-affirming choices.

Try to only write about events that you actually remember, not something that you think or suspect happened. Memories can be slippery, so exercise caution.

If you are getting nowhere after four days of writing on one prompt, then drop that question and try another one. I would also suggest bringing up the topic with a spiritual adviser or mental health professional.

You might find yourself feeling uncomfortable after a writing session. This is normal because you are bringing up thoughts and feelings that you normally would not. I would suggest planning ahead for this by setting up an appointment with a mental health professional, spiritual adviser, or trusted friend; or plan an outing to a park, select an uplifting movie to watch, or engage in a fun activity.

If you find yourself entertaining thoughts of self-harm during the course of thinking about or writing based on these prompts, put this book down and call 911 or the Suicide and Crisis Lifeline, 988.

Eventually you might find it helpful to share your stories with a friend who listens well. This will give you more of a voice and help you become more authentic in everyday life. You will also feel like you have an ally.

At some point, through the writing process or even sharing with another person, you might start to find meaning and purpose in your pain. You will have more perspective and objectivity, and you will feel more complete. You might even be able to reframe the entire journey and integrate it into your life. This will change your life in positive ways. Sometimes this gives our bodies the space and openness to shed illnesses.

Eventually try picking up the threads of your writing to create a coherent story. This includes structure, causal explanation, repetition of themes, a narrative that includes how we felt then and how we feel now, and an awareness of a listener's perspective. Include what sustained you during that time. The more detailed, organized, and lucid our writing is, the greater will be the benefit to our health. Reading out loud what we have written, so it is witnessed by others, can reinforce this process. The goal is a type of writing that is emotionally, psychologically, spiritually, and perhaps even physically healing. You will be creating a space in which you can write stories that tell the truth of your experience. It will make use of your power of imagination and self-expression. It will increase your awareness of yourself as an individual. This ability to re-member the past, speak our truth, imagine the future, and then connect these in a meaningful way, not only heals, it also gives us greater creative power.

DIVE TO THRIVE

At the end of each section is a "Dive to Thrive" option where deeper healing can occur. It involves what social psychologist James Pennebaker calls "expressive writing." He asked study participants to "write about your very deepest thoughts and feelings about an extremely important emotional issue that has affected you and your life. In your writing, I'd like you to really let go and explore your very deepest emotions and thoughts.... The only rule is that once you begin writing, continue to do so until your time is up."[3]

For maximum benefit, he suggests handwriting about a traumatic event for fifteen to twenty minutes per day for three to five days in a row. The goal is to bring up any pain without inhibition, yet also not to let it engulf you. This allows a lot of healing to take place.

Expressive writing can bring up hard, heavy experiences that feel threatening, which is why we usually push them out of everyday awareness. We keep secrets, even from ourselves, to avoid feeling shame. Our concealed knowledge, however, still affects us. It hasn't really gone anywhere. "We are only as sick as our secrets" is a familiar saying to people in recovery from substance use disorder. If our secrets, and the stories we are telling ourselves, are part of what is making us sick, then the antidote is to allow ourselves to encounter these hidden parts of ourselves and rewrite our internal scripts. Telling parts of our histories can unleash our bodies' abilities to heal. We then feel like we have a little more control over our lives.

By doing this within the privacy of our own awareness, we can take a look at what arises, allow the emotions to pass through us, find ways to process the shame, and then let go of the secrets and the shame.

Try to write something new each time you sit down to write, so you can gain more perspectives on the event.

To be effective, this option needs to be vivid, totally honest, and deep. It's not an exercise in complaining or over-analyzing. In fact, sometimes it's the stories we have told ourselves that are what make us sick. If so, these stories need to be expressed and then reframed with meaning. Studies have found that when people described negative emotions excessively—

or very little—there was no improvement in health. To reduce the impact of our negative internal storyteller on our health, we can write about what happened in a way that helps us discover how and why we feel the way we do. The more positive emotions that are included in the narrative, the healthier people become. If the process leads to finding meaning in the events that upset us, we can begin to accept what happened and look for things we learned or gained from the trial. This is where positive outcomes reside. How did the event shape your character? Did it impact how you react in particular ways, and if so, can you begin responding in more thoughtful ways instead? How can you find some peace with what occurred? These types of prompts can assist us with looking forward instead of backward.

When I sat down to do this process, I chose to write for a full 20 minutes straight on a decades-old wound I was still harboring. I wrote directly inside my regular journal to have a record of what occurred.

After I had written steadily for fifteen minutes, I felt complete and wanted to stop. Yet some internal nudge urged me to continue. So I kept moving my pen, adding a couple of repetitious sentences. And then, to my great surprise, treasures poured out of my soul and onto the paper. I received insights and fresh understanding that I'd never found after decades of ruminations and writing about my thoughts and feelings. It seemed like an escape valve had finally opened, and the deepest secrets I had kept from myself found release. I saw a behavior pattern that had led me into decades of difficulties and pain. By pushing past my normal wall, deeper levels of healing brought a lightness into my way of being in the world. Had I stopped when I normally would have felt complete, I would have missed these gems. I could not access these revelations through thinking and exercising my will. I had to bypass normal mental barriers by going around them. Expressive writing distracted my mind and allowed my uninhibited, unfiltered, and unfettered feelings and thoughts to rise up into awareness.

On Day 2, I wrote for another twenty minutes. Again, right at the fifteen-minute mark, I felt complete with writing about the pain and wanted to put down my pen. Recalling how I had pushed through that barrier the previous day and was rewarded with helpful insights, I pushed through again, writing repetitive sentences. And a new insight—this time in the form of a perfect metaphor—arose that fit so well I thought: "Why didn't I think of that before, after decades of trying to describe what happened?" Well, because it had to come from below my normal awareness. The metaphor also felt visceral and, in an odd way, deeply satisfying. Now I could point to the image and say: "That's exactly how it felt!" I didn't have to share it with anyone; my satisfaction came from within.

On Day 3, I again hit the wall at fifteen minutes. It wasn't as firm a barrier this time, and I was able to glide past it with my pen. I saw more fully the life-enhancing lessons I could glean from the painful event and the warning signs I needed to heed as I moved forward. This also felt deeply rewarding.

On Day 4, I just wrote on and on, and inadvertently came across a solution that would help me find more meaning and purpose. That gave me hope and a plan.

Writing in this way does not necessarily lead to any answers, yet if we have the courage to go deeply into our suffering and become present with our own pain, we open ourselves to healing.

If you start to become anxious while writing, just know that this is a signal indicating that you are committed to the process, doing significant work, and growing and changing through your writing. Putting pen to paper allows us to move through the pain from a safe distance. At the same time, it opens a direct pathway from the thoughts and emotions to paper without the intermediary of a keyboard and screen—which can put us in an analytical mode, interfering with our internal processes and potential insights.

Before you start writing in the "Dive to Thrive" processes outlined in this book, be aware that any emotions that arise might last well beyond the writing session. I suggest the following ways to prepare for this:

First, find a mental health professional you can contact in case the writing becomes too stressful. I had a clinical psychologist and a tai chi grandmaster working with me as I journeyed through cancer and beyond. Their wisdom added enormously to my ability to cope and eventually heal.

Second, consider writing on separate sheets of paper so you can shred or burn them as a way to help you let go of the pain.

Third, as you write, try to notice any physical signs that might indicate a need to pause. These can include a drive to eat junk food or use unhealthy substances; excessive sweating; an increased heart rate; a sense of panic; or anything else that signals a high level of stress. If you find yourself in distress, I encourage you to stop and reach out to your mental health professional.

Fourth, you may want to prepare a method for coping with what you discover. Perhaps have some soothing music handy, plan to take a walk, or do some expressive form of art. If possible, have someone prepared to receive a call to discuss your insights.

Fifth, do something afterward that brings you joy as a gift to yourself for your bravery.

I believe expressive writing helped save my life. While undergoing cancer treatment, I wrote in my personal journal quite frequently, sometimes every day. It became a sounding board, a trusted friend, and a valuable aid. Processing my thoughts and feelings in the pages of my journals helped me let go of a lot of longstanding emotional pain. After two years of treatment for end-stage cancer, I went into radical remission. I have been free of any evidence and any treatment for that cancer since 2011.

My hope is you will also enjoy the benefits of writing through cancer.

Sources:

1. *Journal of Clinical Oncology*, Volume 20, Issue 20, October 2002. Randomized, Controlled Trial of Written Emotional Expression and Benefit Finding in Breast Cancer Patients. Annette L. Stanton, Sharon Danoff-Burg, Lisa A. Sworowski, Charlotte A. Collins, Ann D. Branstetter, Alicia Rodriguez-HanleySarah B. Kirk, Jennifer L. Austenfeld from the Department of Psychology, University of Kansas, Lawrence, KS
2. *Journal of Clinical Oncology*, Volume 32, Issue 7, March 1, 2014: Randomized Controlled Trial of Expressive Writing for Patients with

Renal Cell Carcinoma, Kathrin Milbury, Amy Spelman, Christopher Wood, Surena F. Matin, Nizar Tannir, Eric Jonasch, Louis Pisters, Qi Wei, Lorenzo Cohen. All authors: The University of Texas MD Anderson Cancer Center, Houston, TX.

3. Pennebaker, James W. "Writing about Emotional Experiences as a Therapeutic Process." *Psychological Science* Vol. 8, No. 3, May 1997, pg. 162.

1

CONVENTIONAL METHODS

○ ○

DIAGNOSIS

I did not know about this writing process in 2009 when I was diagnosed with highly aggressive end-stage uterine cancer, yet I had been keeping a journal since I was eight years old. After an initial nine-hour surgery, I was hospitalized for nine days. When I got home, I needed to figure out how to manage what was left of my life and go see the nationally rated sarcoma specialists that my sister had found for me.

I felt completely overwhelmed.

It was six weeks before I finally sat down to write about what was happening inside me: "Why have I hardly even cried? Hardly felt anything? Am I numb to it all? Part of me certainly wants to just let go and check out of life. I don't want to go through these chemotherapy treatments. And even if I get well, I still must deal with all my problems."

Soon after, I read Louise Hay's book, *You Can Heal Your Life*, and did more investigative writing. "The bottom line in all dis-ease is a sense that 'I'm not good enough.' Yes, I've unknowingly held this belief from the womb. That's the feeling of not being loved, wanted, or even seen … and a feeling of 'I don't deserve.' This sense probably arose because I was the fourth child born in less than six years, and my mother was, understandably, completely exhausted. It is the root of many of my issues with other people. It was reflected in my deferring to others because I did not value my own thoughts and opinions enough."

I had dug around and discovered one of the roots of my illness. It gave me a starting point for the road to regaining my health and letting go of disease. I came to understand that the cancer was the kick in the pants I needed to get into my body, feel my emotions, and deeply heal my past. It had a purpose for me, and I had a mission to accomplish if I wanted to stay alive.

PROMPTS TO GET YOU STARTED:

Cancer?! What the heck…

I can't believe this is happening!

Why me?

Tests, doctors, more tests, more doctors…

Test results drive me crazy!

What are my conventional treatment options? What are the potential benefits and drawbacks for each of them?

How do I plan to be assertive with my treatment team to make sure I get honest and complete answers?

What treatment options do I believe are best for me?

What is going to happen to me?

What is going to happen to my loved ones?

These are the things that scare me the most…

I was really angry when…

Why aren't they…

Why didn't I…

Please! Won't you just…

I really hate…

I feel like…

What's most important to me today?

What do I need right now from my support system?

What do I need right now from myself?

What will I do to get my needs met?

If the cancer could talk to me, what would it say?

If I could talk directly to the cancer, what would I say?

What is something I can feel good about right now?

How can I reframe this diagnosis in a positive way?

Do I believe I can go into remission? If yes, what am I doing to move in that direction? If not, how can I work toward having hope?

What happiness and good fortune might be lurking within my diagnosis?

How have my values changed since getting the diagnosis?

What have I learned about myself since getting the diagnosis?

MOVING DEEPER:

What is my diagnosis story?

What sustained me through the first few weeks and months? How do I feel now?

What new attitudes have I developed since the diagnosis?

How else have I changed after getting this diagnosis?

How did this help me grow emotionally, psychologically, spiritually?

What will a healthy future look like for me? What will it include?

What meaning and purpose can I find in this diagnosis?

DIVE TO THRIVE:

What are my very deepest thoughts and feelings about the diagnosis? How has it affected me as a person as well as affected my life? How did the event shape my character? Did it impact how I react in particular ways, and if so, how can I begin responding in more thoughtful ways instead? How can I find some peace with what occurred?

CHEMOTHERAPY

When I was sixteen months old, I would grab a handful of my hair, twist it, and pull it out. Of course, this greatly distressed my mother, who had my hair cut very short. Then she added a cap with a throat strap so I couldn't pull the cap off. Her method broke the habit but did not get at the root cause.

After the cancer diagnosis, I discussed my hair-pulling with my psychotherapist, who suggested I was pulling out my hair as a distraction from a stressful situation.

Well, end-stage cancer was also stressful. To top it off, I was told I would lose my hair within three weeks of starting chemotherapy. I got my hair cut really short to manage it when it would start falling out, just like it was when I was sixteen months old, though I didn't realize it at the time.

I sat down with a photo of my 16-month-old self to emotionally re-enter my experience as a toddler. I imitated sucking my thumb, with my left fingers curled over my nose and my right hand behind my right ear, twirling my hair.

Oh, that felt so familiar, so comfortable, so soothing.

As an adult writing, I engaged that emotional landscape and recognized anxiety—a mood created by thinking about something. Perhaps I had been "thinking," as much as a toddler could, to avoid feeling the fear in my body. So, I went into the fear and allowed my body to feel it.

As it turned out, after starting chemotherapy at age forty-eight, I did not lose my hair in twenty-one days. It took twenty-one months of chemotherapy.

When I finally did lose my hair, it happened all at once and was physically painful. I was reliving what I had done to myself as a child, yet it was a one-off event, and I still had plenty of hair left on my scalp when the chemo deed was done.

I don't imagine a lot of people pulled out their hair as toddlers, yet there might have been another difficult, high-stress situation that left you feeling like you were symbolically pulling out your hair. It might be something worth exploring.

PROMPTS TO GET YOU STARTED:

OMG, chemotherapy?

What is going to happen to me?

These are the things that scare me the most…

I really hate…

I am really angry about…

I feel like…

How can I best prepare for chemotherapy?

How can I reframe chemotherapy as a faithful friend whose wounds can heal, as a method for ridding my body of evil, and to honor my drive toward life?

How can I imagine the chemotherapy working inside my body?

What can I do to turn my chemotherapy treatment session into something I enjoy?

What resources do I have to make sure my needs are met?

What specific needs do I have right now, and who can I ask for help to get them met?

What can I do to keep some awareness of what is happening inside my body even during the discomfort of treatment?

What does it feel like to be my heart, be my hands, be my feet, be my belly, be my intestines during the chemotherapy die-off phase?

What can I do to relax more and get more rest so my body can recover?

Am I whining and complaining too much? If so, how can I turn that around?

How do I feel about losing my hair? How does it affect my view of myself?

How do I feel about other people who have luxurious hair when mine has to be shaved off?
How does it feel to be bald?

How do I feel about being bald around family? Friends? Strangers? If I feel different with different people, what causes those differences?

How do I feel when I push the limits of my comfort levels while I am out in public with a bald head?

How does being bald bring out more of my inner beauty? Which of my best three qualities are now shining through the brightest?

How do I feel about my hair regrowing? How do I feel about its texture and color?

In what ways can I approach the cancer globally—changing the environment within my body by changing my life—while acting locally to take out the cells that are growing too fast?

Am I thinking about quitting chemotherapy? If so, how have others in a similar situation survived, both with and without continued infusions? What other options did they choose, and how did they fare? How does that leave me feeling?

What else can be done so I receive the support and assistance I need if I decide to continue with chemotherapy?

What options do I have if chemotherapy stops working? How do I feel about them?

How do I feel about getting off chemotherapy? How am I managing my doubts and insecurities?

After chemotherapy ends, what can I do to continue in a positive direction? What complementary therapies should I consider?
How can I be on the alert for post-chemotherapy scams since this is a time of greater vulnerability?

Now that I have been through chemotherapy, what foods can I enjoy? Which fragrances?

What is something I can feel good about right now?

MOVING DEEPER:

What is my chemotherapy story? What sustained me through the treatments? What was hardest and how did I cope? What turned out to be easier than I expected?

How did chemotherapy help me grow emotionally, psychologically, spiritually?

What new attitudes have I developed because I have endured chemotherapy?

What meaning and purpose can I find as a result of the chemotherapy experience?

DIVE TO THRIVE:

Think about a painful experience caused by chemotherapy. What are my very deepest thoughts and feelings about it? How has it affected me as a person as well as affected my life? How did the event shape my character? Did it impact how I react in particular ways, and if so, how can I begin responding in more thoughtful ways instead? How can I find some peace with what occurred?

SURGERY

After two years of chemotherapy, my scan results came in. I had yet another nodule, this time more than half an inch in diameter, sitting on the pulmonary vein next to my heart. And I had run out of effective chemotherapy options.

My thoughts were churning, churning, churning. So, I sat down to write.

Rage—Why won't the cancer STOP?
Terror—I'm definitely going to die!
Loss—I will never get my life back.
Grief—My life is over.
Victim—There's nothing I can do.
Powerlessness—The trap door underneath me has opened and I'm falling through.
Despair—Why bother even trying? It's hopeless.

At the same time, my marriage was in crisis, my 15-year-old son was getting drunk, and my father's dementia was worsening.

What to do, what to do? Everything lay in shambles.

My friend Kathryn suggested I imagine placing all the junk in my body into that tumor so it would leave when the surgeon took out the tumor. Why not? So, I did that.

I had the surgery, and during my 6-week post-operation checkup with a nurse practitioner, she told me the half-inch nodule had, in five weeks, grown to 2.5 inches.

And yet, the surgery was successful. When combined with all my complementary and integrative treatments, I entered into radical remission, remaining free of evidence of the sarcoma and free of its medical treatment.

PROMPTS TO GET YOU STARTED:

OMG, surgery?

What is going to happen to me?

These are the things that scare me the most...

I really hate ...

I am really angry about...

I feel like...

Where am I holding tension in my body? How does it feel to stay with the tension until it relaxes on its own? In what ways can I become soft and yielding toward the procedure?

What do I need right now from my support system?

What do I need right now from myself?

What is something I can feel good about right now?

How can I reframe surgery? As a faithful friend that is directly removing unhealthy body parts? As a way to honor my drive toward life?

How can I best prepare for surgery?

What will I need after surgery, and how will I get those needs met? Who can I ask for help, even with the small things?

What can I do to reduce the need for pain medications after surgery?

What can I do to relax more and get more rest so my body can recover?

Am I whining and complaining too much? If so, how can I turn that around?
What can I do to continue in a positive direction? What complementary therapies should I consider?

If I were to use my scar as a basis for a tattoo, what image would I place there?

How do I feel about living without a whole body when I am around family? Friends? Strangers? If I feel different with different people, what causes those differences?

If an obvious part of my body is missing, how do I feel when I push the limits of my comfort levels when out in public?

How does being without a certain part of my body bring out more of my inner beauty? Which of my best three qualities are shining through the brightest?

What new attitudes, such as compassion, have I developed because of the surgery?

MOVING DEEPER:

When living with a stomach tube, think about the Hindu god Ganesh, who is known for removing obstacles. What unnecessary emotional baggage am I carrying around? What obstacles are standing in the way of my healing? What can I do about each of them?

The late Jungian psychoanalyst Marion Woodman recorded her cancer experiences in *Bone: Dying into Life*. She brilliantly connected the words scarred->scared->sacred. How can I view my surgery as a sacrifice in preparation for the next step in my inner development? In my outer life?

What is my surgery story? What sustained me during and after the surgery? What meaning and purpose can I find as a result of the surgical experience?

How did the surgery help me grow emotionally, psychologically, spiritually?

DIVE TO THRIVE:

Think about the most traumatic experience you have had that was caused by surgery, or a previous loss of a body part. What are my very deepest thoughts and feelings about it? How has it affected me as a person as well as affected my life? How did the event shape my character? Did it impact how I react in particular ways, and if so, how can I begin responding in more thoughtful ways instead? How can I find some peace with what occurred?

RADIATION

While I have not been treated with radiation, I did feel the burn of several types of chemotherapy. Among them was doxorubicin (Adriamycin), nicknamed the Red Devil. These drugs spread a dark, prickly, uncomfortable sensation throughout my body and pretty much burned through my digestive system for a few days during each cycle. Among the side-effects were painful mouth sores, skin over-sensitivity, and burning stools. My hands and feet looked burned—red and sore and even blistery.

I would follow the die-off phase with Tai Chi Grandmaster Vincent J. Lasorso's "Bone Marrow Healing" visualization. During this recording, he would suggest that I feel my bones lighting up—not seeing in my mind's eye, but instead feeling into my bones. The process started at my feet and moved up my body, so my whole skeleton would feel a tender vibration when I finished.

Later, as I wrote about it, I discovered something. I had the negative experience of the burning sensation of every cell in my body juxtaposed by the positive experience of feeling my bones lighting up. This gradually extended into my ability to feel the rest of the cells in my body lighting up.

As Lasorso later pointed out to me, without the dark, burning, prickling of chemotherapy, this wonderful awakening inside my cells might never have happened.

PROMPTS TO GET YOU STARTED:

OMG, radiation? What the...

I can't believe it!

What is going to happen to me?

These are the things that scare me the most...

I really hate...

I am really angry about...

I feel like...

Where am I holding tension in my body? How does it feel to stay with the tension until it relaxes on its own? In what ways can I become soft and yielding toward the procedures?

How can I best prepare for radiation?

What do I need right now from my support system?

What do I need right now from myself?

What will I do to get my needs met?

What is something I can feel good about right now?

How can I reframe radiation in a positive way?

MOVING DEEPER:

What is my radiation story? What did I feel when initially told I could benefit from radiation? How do I feel now? What sustained me through the first few weeks and months?

How have I changed after getting the radiation treatments?

How did this treatment help me grow emotionally, psychologically, spiritually?

What meaning and purpose can I find in the results of the radiation treatments?

What new attitudes have I developed because of the radiation treatments?

What will a healthy future look like for me? What will it include?

DIVE TO THRIVE:

What are my very deepest thoughts and feelings about the radiation treatments? How has this experience affected me as a person as well as affected my life? How did the event shape my character? Did it impact how I react in particular ways, and if so, how can I begin responding in more thoughtful ways instead? How can I find some peace with what occurred?

2

CONGRUENT CARE

O O

Fear imprisoned me, and the prospect of a painful death created abject terror in my body. There was no acceptance and no freedom in my vocabulary because the cancer was relentless, month after month, treatment cycle after treatment cycle.

To deal with the potential of an agonizing death, I was reminded of the story in Judges 11 of the Jewish Bible about the daughter of Jephthah. Her father made a foolish vow to the Divine to make a burnt offering of the first thing to meet him after returning home from a war victory. Upon arriving at his house after winning, the first thing to greet him was his joyful daughter, who was singing and dancing. The father insisted on keeping the promise even when it involved murdering an innocent victim. The daughter bowed to his will.

I felt incensed when I read this story. Not only was the woman never given the dignity of a name, but no angel appeared with a ram at the last moment to save her from an agonizing death (as it did for Isaac in the Jewish book of Genesis).

This daughter understood herself well enough to relish the joy of music and dance. She loved her father. She knew she needed time to prepare for her demise and required support—so she asked for what she needed.

With great courage, she spent two months in retreat, contemplating her impending agony. She must have felt rage, terror, grief, and powerlessness during those two months. She did not run away from fulfilling her role. She faced it with grace. She mourned the things she would never experience in life.

I sat down and wrote about her situation, and mine. Where is the purpose behind such tragic, senseless deaths? It seems totally insane. Yet the Spirit allowed it to happen. The daughter showed a profound acceptance of "things as they are." Not many types of death are worse than being burned alive. She did not cajole, bargain, try to influence or control, give up, or deny the situation.

She must have died in great equanimity with radiant acceptance. I had much yet to learn from her example.

I came to understand that sometimes illness and death are part of the ultimate plan. The Spirit walks and weeps with us and can offer us strength and courage even as we pass into the next existence.

We do not always understand the circumstances of our lives and why things happen as they do. Sometimes simply accepting things as they are is the best solution, along with learning to be, to breathe into the moment, and to allow.

I needed to learn to love myself and to experience myself as the Spirit experiences me—whole, and healthy, and healed. Whether that means I would be physically cured or not was not up to me. Through my questioning and writing, I was moving closer to release into freedom, into equanimity, and into radiant acquiescence. By facing this, I could also face the end-of-life questions I needed to address.

PROMPTS TO GET YOU STARTED:

Are my affairs in order? If not, who can I call for a referral?

If my life goes on the line, how do I want to be treated by the medical community? What do I need to do to ensure I have a health care power of attorney in place who will make health care decisions for me if I no longer can for myself?

Under what circumstances do I want to be kept on life support?

Do I want the use of cardio-pulmonary resuscitation?

Who do I want to handle financial matters for me if I become unable? How do I want them handled?

What do I want in my Living Will? Do I want both water and nutrition during the final stages of illness, or if a surgery goes wrong?

How do I want to approach death, should it become inevitable?

If I should pass,
Who do I want to represent me and carry out my wishes?
What will this person be enabled to do?
Who do I want to inherit my belongings?
When and how do I want my property distributed?
Who do I want to become the legal guardians for any minor children?

MOVING DEEPER:

Sometimes we must face and accept death before we discover how we want to live. Right now, am I truly living my life? How can I remember who I truly am?

Who am I, really?

How has cancer affected me as a person as well as affected my life?

DIVE TO THRIVE:

What are my very deepest thoughts and feelings about losing my life? How can I find some peace with this?

3

COMPLEMENTARY THERAPIES

o o

As you approach each of these sections, start with the easier prompts, and work your way toward being able to Move Deeper and then finally Dive to Thrive. The gold at the end can be worth the journey.

LET FOOD BE YOUR MEDICINE

When I was in grade school, my father left his military career and started working on his doctorate. We moved into a brand-new house and had two big brand-new cars to accommodate our family of seven. My mother tried her hand at real estate, but after a year she still had not sold a single home. So, money was pretty tight.

While we always had food on the table, it was not always appetizing. And living in a military family, the consequences for not following the rules were severe. I could not get up from the table until I had finished what was put on my plate... and if, perchance, I did not finish eating and went straight to bed instead, whatever I did not consume was saved for the next meal, and the next meal, and the next... so I pretty much had to eat what was put in front of me. These indigestibles included tall glasses of reconstituted powdered milk that my siblings labelled "sludge;" very dense, nasty-tasting old bread from the commissary that we called "lead bread;" and organ meats like liver, kidneys, and the coup de grâce, slimy pork brains. Gag.

After my cancer diagnosis, I started making green smoothies every day. Because at this point cancer was also eating at the finances, I tried to find the least expensive ways to get my dark leafies. I ended up settling mostly on blanched weeds from the yard. Then I would add whatever I didn't want to eat—water hyssop for brain health; lion's mane powder for memory; dandelion stems for bone health; red clover blossoms for calcium; fermented purslane for omega-3s… the list went on. The mix got so bitter I found myself, once again, gagging as I tried to make this new style of sludgy slide down my throat.

I decided it was time to Dive to Thrive.

To my surprise, I realized I had been living out a compulsion to repeat the food torture my parents had inflicted on me. I uncovered anger both at them and at myself, so I spent some time allowing my body to shake it out.

And then I realized: Oh, this is why people pop pills. And I asked myself: why am I torturing myself so much that I gagged? Was I really digesting the nutrients if I could barely keep the sludgies down?

I knew it was time for a change. Why not blanch broccoli, kale, or cabbage, then put them into my high-speed blender with a nourishing bone broth and some sprouted cooked barley? I could add some healthy fat and then sip with enjoyment! And during the summer, I could grow more mint and blend that with cocoa powder and add a healthy sweetener. Yummy!

PROMPTS TO GET YOU STARTED:

What types of healthy foods do I find appealing and attractive? Raw veggies or soups and stews? Fish or beef or beans? Spicy or bland foods? How do I prefer them to be prepared?

What can I do to increase the number of colors of my produce each day to achieve the rainbow ideal?

How do different types of food affect how my body feels?
Meat?
Dairy?
Grains?
Beans?
Nuts?

How does my body feel after each meal? What about for the next several hours? What kind of end-product does my body produce?

In what ways can I improve my choices with:
Produce?
Grains?
Beans?
Fish and/or Meat?
Dairy?

How do I feel about altering my diet to improve my chances of survival?

MOVING DEEPER:

What stories do I tell myself about the foods I choose to eat or avoid? How can I turn those stories into something positive?

DIVE TO THRIVE:

What are my deepest thoughts and feelings about a traumatic event or long-term stress regarding food? What happened? What were my thoughts and feelings about it then? How do I feel about it now? What do I choose to learn from the experience? How has my perspective changed? How did the event shape my character? Did it impact how I react in particular ways, and if so, how can I begin responding in more thoughtful ways instead? How can I find some peace with what occurred?

MINDING THE BODY

One morning I woke up with a feeling of sorrow and powerlessness. In my heart sat a mysterious heaviness and physical pain. I allowed the uncomfortable sensations to be what they were, just feeling them without thinking about them. I did not know what they were about, and I did not seek understanding at that point.

Later I wrote in my journal about feeling helpless, powerless, and victimized. I asked my intuition, "What is the source for these sensations?"

I traced back through my life as far back as memory and my pen could take me. Then a door opened up inside me. I recalled being told that when I was a toddler, I was shoved down a flight of stairs. I had been bullied and victimized. Because I did not have any physical injuries from it, nothing much was done about it.

Suddenly I realized that such an incident at so young an age would most likely lead to far-reaching repercussions. This incident needed further exploration.

What had I experienced while tumbling helplessly down a flight of stairs?

Terror. Powerlessness. Helplessness.

I sat down in a chair to go deeply into those sensations of falling. Immediately my body remembered. I screamed and shook all over, off and on, for ninety minutes. My body also let go of a great deal of heat. Finally, exhausted, I knew I had released some deep wounds.

As I returned to writing in my journal, I realized that my cells had frozen in time, carrying this trauma like armor all through my life. My cells had been perpetually caught in the drama, always bracing for yet another impact, and had never unclenched all the way. Even though my conscious mind was unconscious of the event, my body knew and remembered.

Because my body had kept itself armored, I somehow attracted more bullies throughout my life. Letting go of the armor and softening the bracing would allow easier blood flow in my body, more relaxation, and an opportunity for developing more enjoyable relationships with others.

PROMPTS TO GET YOU STARTED:

What did I really love doing as a child but don't really do anymore? What is stopping me from doing those activities now, and what would happen if I did them? In what ways can I replicate those now in ways that are fun and don't interfere with my treatments?

What do I now love doing most, and how can I spend more time doing that?

What can I create right now?

Is my daily routine serving my movement toward greater health? Does anything need an adjustment?

Do my living conditions depress me or excite me? Are there other options I can explore?

Does my job enliven or depress me? If it depresses me, what can I do to remedy the situation?

What in my physical environment is interfering with my ability to heal? What can I do about it?

What do I still want to experience in my life?

Where am I holding tension in my body? How does it feel to stay with the tension until it relaxes on its own?

What does my cancer look like today?

How can I live more in the present moment, from the inside out?

What can I do to increase the amount of time I do deep breathing each day?

Without defining, using language, or judging, how does my body feel right now, on the inside?

How can I raise my awareness of what I am feeling inside my body?

If I try to let go of an expectation, how does my body respond?

How does the word "acceptance" feel in my body?

How can I move toward accepting my body as it is now?

How can I nurture myself today?

What would my behavior look like if I altered it in a healthier direction? How can I pull that new sense of well-being into myself? How would that feel?

If I were to have a dialogue with my body that involved a back-and-forth conversation, how would it read?

If I were to pretend that my body is more like a fountain of light than a sculpture of stone, what kind of shift could I make to both renew my physical body and view myself as in(a)curable state of being?

Author Deepak Chopra, MD, suggests lying on one's bed before going to sleep and simply allowing the body and lungs to let out sighs, in whatever way feels best, for about ten minutes. This process allows the body to let go of stored or blocked energy. When I try this method, what happens, and how do I feel about it?

MOVING DEEPER:

What have I learned about my body since my diagnosis?

What is the symbolism of the bodily location of my cancer? What message might it have for me?

At the end of the 1939 movie "The Wizard of Oz" (produced by Metro-Goldwyn-Mayer), Glinda stands next to Dorothy and says, "You have always had the power within you." The Christian gospels tell how Jesus could feel healing energy pass out of his body into others' bodies (Mark 5:30), and that we could do more than he (John 14:12). The Islamic Qur'an mentions believers who have "light streaming before them and by their right hands" (Sura 57:12, and repeated in Sura 66:8, Thomas Cleary translation). That means we have that potential healing energy in our own bodies. We are our own greatest healers. What options can I access for learning how to heal my own body? What can I do to help myself access this power?

DIVE TO THRIVE:

What are my very deepest thoughts and feelings about an ongoing bad childhood situation I survived? What happened? What were my thoughts and feelings about it then? What sort of expectations did my child-self form because of it? How do I feel about it now? What do I choose to learn from the experience? How has my perspective changed? How did the event shape my character? Did it impact how I react in particular ways, and if so, how can I begin responding in more thoughtful ways instead? How can I find some peace with what occurred?

MAPPING THE EMOTIONS

Soon after I was diagnosed with highly aggressive end-stage cancer, I picked up Louise Hay's book, *You Can Heal Your Life*. She said the bottom line for all dis-ease is "I'm not good enough." I wrote in my journal about this sense—for me it seemed to be shame about even existing. While I knew I was loved, I did not feel that love because it was covered over by shame. I did not feel wanted or even seen, which were childhood misperceptions of my situation.

As I wrote, I uncovered another aspect to my shame—that I did not deserve good things. Because of this unconscious attitude, I deferred to what others wanted, let people bully me, and did not ask for what I needed.

Now that I could literally see the unhelpful attitudes I had unconsciously harbored, I could set the record straight, at least mentally. I knew in my mind that I was loved; that I was good enough, just because I was human; and that I deserved good things, including regaining my health. I could begin asking for the things I needed and make myself my priority.

Later I would learn how to feel my emotions without censoring, judging, or analyzing them. Those concepts are included in the Mapping the Emotions section of the book *Thriver Soup: A Feast for Living Consciously During the Cancer Journey*. But first I had to get my thoughts out of the way, which allowed me to get in touch with my emotions. I used writing sessions to process what was going on in my head, which gave me more freedom to feel them in my body.

PROMPTS TO GET YOU STARTED:

Right now, in this moment, what am I feeling?

What makes me the angriest? How does that anger feel within my body? Where do I feel it most strongly?

What scares me the most? How does that feel within my body?

Where do I feel my fear the most strongly? How are those fears holding me back?

What am I afraid to admit to myself?

What am I the most afraid of losing, and what would I truly lose if I lost it? How does that fear feel within my body? Where do I feel it most strongly?

In what ways am I afraid to die?

In what ways am I afraid to live?

What are my greatest fears about giving control over to the Divine?

What has caused deep hurt in my life?

What has caused deep sorrow in my life?

What unhealed griefs do I still have?

What does grief feel like in my body?

Cancer leaves us feeling powerless. What can I do to regain some sense of power in my life?

What else causes me to feel powerless? How does that feel within my body? Where do I feel it most strongly?

What is it like in my body when I feel hopelessness?

Under what circumstances do I feel shame? How does that shame feel inside my body? Where do I feel it most strongly? With whom can I safely share this sense of shame?
What is it like in my body when I feel emptiness?

What is it like in my body when I feel loneliness?

What are my deepest yearnings?

What pulls at my energy, drags me down, or makes me feel bad? Do these parts of my life serve me? If not, why am I still hanging on to them? What needs to go? What steps do I need to take to let them go?

What emotional patterns might have contributed to the rise of the disease? How can I shift those patterns?

When an emotion arises for me, what do I do with it?

What unexpressed feelings do I still have?

How will I feel if I put forth my best efforts to survive? To learn what I can and apply it? How will I feel if I do not?

What would happen if I reframed the purpose of the illness as an invitation to learn how to open my heart?

Have I really been living my life, or have I just been getting through life? How do I feel about that?

How do I feel about the privilege of growing old?

What creative pursuits would I like to incorporate into my life right now? How can I go about doing that?

How can I increase my level of contentment with life?

What would be fun to do right now?

What would be pleasant to do right now?

What would bring me happiness right now?
What do I love most about myself?

What brings me joy? How can I create circumstances that inspire joy for me?

Laughter is good medicine. What comedies can I enjoy reading, listening to, or watching?

What opens my heart?

What makes my heart sing?

What does my heart want me to do today?

How can I use cancer as an invitation to open my heart more fully to deeply experience my connection with myself, with others, and with the Spirit?

Who do I know that exudes joy, peace, and love? How can I emulate that in my life? How can I feel those in my body?

MOVING DEEPER:

What inner conflicts might I have about regaining my health? What feelings emerge from my awareness of this conflict? How can I resolve them? (For me, I gained the realization that a part of me did not want to get well because then my disability checks and health insurance would end. It created an uncomfortable inner conflict I knew I needed to resolve.)

What different choices would I make if I knew I would die tomorrow? In a week, a month, or a year? How can I bring my outer choices into alignment with my inner desires? How does that feel when accomplished?[1]

When the mind is still like water in a calm pond (a goal of meditation), one can look into the depths and see cast-off thoughts and emotions lying at the bottom. What is at the lowest point of my metaphorical mind that is longing for my attention?[2]

What emotion has troubled me all my life? What is the root cause? What can I do about the root cause to free myself?

DIVE TO THRIVE:

What are my very deepest thoughts and feelings about a traumatic event that affected me emotionally? What happened? What were my thoughts and feelings about it then? How do I feel about it now? What do I choose to learn from the experience? How has my perspective changed? How did the event shape my character? Did it impact how I react in particular ways, and if so, how can I begin responding in more thoughtful ways instead? How can I find some peace with what occurred?

Sources:

1. Siegel, Bernie S. *Love, Medicine, & Miracles: Lessons Learned About Self-healing from a Surgeon's Experience with Exceptional Patients.* New York: Harper & Row, 1986:96, 97.
2. Markova, Dawna. *I Will Not Die an Unlived Life: Reclaiming Purpose and Passion.* San Francisco: Conari Press, 2000: 38.

MENDING THE MIND

One day I read about word vows that we sometimes make. I looked at my life and saw yet another negative pattern in my relationships, so I questioned if I had ever made a word vow.

I began to write, exploring the issue with my pen. I was shocked to realize I had made a vow while a teenager at a time when I had been anxious, and that promise had negatively influenced my entire adult life.

As I wrote, I ended up with a list of eleven beliefs I had developed and lived by as a result of the one anxiety-based vow: "I'll never... I will always... I can't...". It produced problems of shame, self-pity, and negative pride throughout my adult life. These, in an odd way, "proved" that my anxiety was valid, and I had the little payoff of being "right" to make the vow.

Oh, crap.

I wanted, instead, to cultivate peace, love, and joy.

As I sat with the originating fear, it quickly dissipated—it was grounded in a false idea about religion that I had well outgrown. I became disgusted with the pain and misery I had caused myself. This led to anger at a family member. My knee-jerk reaction was to want to blame, a mind-based way of avoiding the anger I felt. I stopped writing and allowed the anger to rise and move around in my body until it dissipated. Then I saw that I was the one responsible for continuing the pattern and the pain; no one else.

I curled into a fetal position to continue feeling the emotions. After they finally lifted, I asked my inner guidance for help with letting go of the vow and resulting beliefs. Then I saw, in my mind's eye, a scroll of parchment paper with the vow written on it. It was rolled up and tied with a velvety red ribbon and handed to me. In front of me there appeared a limestone altar with a fire burning on top. I placed the sheet into the flames and watched it burn up.

It was finished. The contract was now null and void. I had freed myself from my own foolishness.

PROMPTS TO GET YOU STARTED:

If I had a pet that was diagnosed with cancer, would I blame the pet? Why or why not?

In what ways do I blame myself? Where within my body do I feel it most strongly?

When I am anxious, what does my body do?

I have never talked about this...

The worst lie I ever told...

The meanest thing I ever did...

There is a story I have never shared with someone and now here it is...

My greatest weakness is... and this is how I will work to do better despite this weakness...

What thought patterns might have contributed to the rise of the disease? How can I shift those patterns?

What unresolved conflicts do I still have?

Did I make a word vow at some point that needs to be cleared away?

Am I allowing things to be done to me or am I taking my life into my own hands and putting forth whatever effort is necessary to regain my health?

In what ways would I prefer not to heal? What am I not willing to do?

What is weighing on my mind right now?

What regrets am I likely to have if I continue on my current path?

How can I switch paths to avoid regrets?

In what ways have I been living with misery? How can I resurrect the desire to live?

What would happen if I let go of the need to control the outcome of my health crisis?

Who do I resent? What is the cost to me of giving up my resentment? What can I do to start a forgiveness process regarding that person?

Who else do I need to forgive? How can I move toward being willing to forgive?

What do I need to forgive about myself?

What are my doubts, and how can I manage them in healthy ways?

What do I find confusing?

What scripts does my mind review over and over, like bad newsreels? How can I redirect my thinking, and what would I prefer to be doing with my thoughts?

How can I let go of the expectation that I would live a happy, healthy life?

What are the possible reasons the disease took hold in my body?

Is it possible I was allowing the cancer to continue? If so, in what ways?

Do I have an internal voice that judges and/or shames me? What role has it played in my life? What does it want from me? What were the little payouts it gave me?

What are my three biggest regrets? What can I do about them to rectify the situations?

In what ways has cancer relieved stress for me? How can I continue that trend?

What would my life be like if I viewed the cancer experience as a push on the pause button of my life so I could hit "refresh" and start over as a whole new person?

Which am I more likely to do: Bitch by focusing on the negative? Or fight by doing everything I can to live? What percentage of the time do I do them when thinking? When talking with or writing to others?

If I choose to end an unhealthy situation, how do I want to grow through the process of ending it? How will I grow in integrity?

How do I let go of the need to control the results of my treatments?

What did I used to believe that no longer serves me?

How am I going to approach the dis-ease from here on out?

Is there a life-altering decision that could help me find my way back to health?

Do I really want to live or not? If so, for what reasons—for me and not for others?

How am I going to shift from being a cancer victim to a cancer victor?

Do I believe I have a set expiration point? How does that affect my daily and long-term choices?

How do I balance living life while preparing for death?

What beliefs are holding me back?

What will "success" look like for me?

What has been missing from my life that I now can add to it?

What can I do today to get my needs met?

Am I still going about my life as if nothing has happened, or am I using cancer as a motivator to shed my old, unhelpful ways of being and doing?

What aspects of my life need to be inspected more deeply to see if change needs to be enacted?

How serious am I about healing my life?

What makes me feel glad to be alive? How can I make more of that happen?

What truth have I not admitted to myself? How can I face it?

How can I improve the way I treat myself, talk to myself, and talk about myself?

What is something I really want? If it happened, what would it look like? Feel like? Sound like? Smell like? Taste like?

What do I currently do to express gratitude to myself, others, and the Divine? What more can I reasonably do?

If I am given a new lease on life for an extended time, what would I focus on doing? How would I alter my inner life? What is keeping me from doing those now?

Today I am grateful because...

I really hope...

I would be happier with myself if I...

I want to be more...

My greatest strength is…

How can I be more compassionate with myself?

What can I do to increase my level of confidence?

In what ways can I be more authentic?

What needs to change for me to truly live?

In what ways do I want my life healed?

What would it take for me to fully participate in regaining my health?

What steps can I take today to remove all obstacles to healing my life, whatever the results are for my body?

How can I flip cancer from a foe into a source of deep healing and regeneration?

What might be keeping me from fully accepting healing?

How can I increase my ability to trust in the processes of life for my healing and perhaps even a cure?

What are my reasons for living?

How can I extend more kindness to myself?

What was something difficult I was able to overcome? How did I overcome it?

How can I most easily reduce stress in my life?

What is my true passion and life purpose? How can I arouse that vocation within myself?

How can I develop an unreserved, positive self-adoration and be reborn?

What would a love letter to myself say about all the beauty within my soul and all the kind things I have done for myself and others?

If I stayed true at all times to my deepest, most authentic self, what would I change in my life? How can I begin moving in that direction?

If I fully accepted and loved myself, how would I be different from how I am now? How can I make that happen?

How can I use cancer as an initiation into a more profound manifestation of inner wisdom?

What gifts have I given myself after the cancer diagnosis? What gifts have I given others because of the cancer?

What special treatment or gifts do I receive because I have cancer? Do I feel attached to these, enough to avoid getting well?

What gifts do I have that I was born to offer the world? What am I doing to help bring those to light and share them with others?

What unfinished business do I still have—things to try, to give, or to learn?

Am I who I want to be? If not, what can I do to change myself?

Am I proud of my life? If not, what can I do to change it?

When I get beyond cancer treatment, who do I want my new self to be? What qualities do I want to possess?

What do I still want to learn?

What is my "happily ever-after" fairy-tale ending for my personal story?

MOVING DEEPER:

According to Lazaris, who speaks through Jach Pursel, children make shame-based contracts with adults to stop pain and survive.

1. The child becomes a clone of a parent or defies the parent and becomes his or her opposite.
2. The child chooses to never grow up, to always seek the parent's approval, to live out the parent's dreams, or to be perfect.
3. The child becomes an abuser to justify the abuse already received; metes out punishment; chooses never to have a negative impact on others; chooses never to admit to being wrong; or chooses not to feel.
4. The child develops an intense connection with the parental figure through cords connecting their energy centers (a symbolic representation of any contract). Then the child surrenders individuality.[1]

If any of these match my experiences, how might I heal?

Source:

1. https://www.lazaris.com/shop-product/lazaris-series/evenings-with-lazaris/ending-shame-part-ii-psychic-contracts-of-pain/ retrieved 5/23/2015.

DIVE TO THRIVE:

What are my very deepest thoughts and feelings about a traumatic event that strongly affected my thought processes and attitudes? What happened? What were my thoughts and feelings about it then? How do I feel about it now? Did it give rise to resentment, anxiety, or a victim or martyr mentality? What do I choose to learn from the experience? How has my perspective changed? How did the event shape my character?

Did it impact how I react in particular ways, and if so, how can I begin responding in more thoughtful ways instead? How can I find some peace with what occurred?

IT TAKES A VILLAGE

If, as I had read in several places, resentments lie underneath many cancer diagnoses, then I needed to clear them out. Resentment is what happens when we think about what "makes" us angry. And I had a lot of unprocessed anger.

I asked my intuition for guidance. It responded by providing a new name every morning of someone else I needed to forgive. Often it involved a situation in which I was bullied. *Ask and you shall receive*, I thought with chagrin.

I would write out the problem for as long as I needed to, stopping occasionally to feel the emotions as sensations in my body. Gradually, I would move into forgiveness.

After a couple of weeks, I homed in on a more recent incident. I wrote and wrote about what she had done to hurt me, what I was angry about, and how she had bullied me.

As I moved into asking myself if her bullying behavior was part of a larger pattern in my life, I had a sudden insight. I had heard for decades that "like attracts like." I had heard for decades about how humans repress what they don't like about themselves and then see those same characteristics in others. Now, for the first time, those concepts truly made sense. I saw them operating inside of me. This woman had bullied me because I was a bully.

Who, me? A bully? No way! I am a "nice" person. I didn't go around bullying people!

But then I thought about the phrase, "like attracts like." I had attracted many bullies into my life because I was a bully. I had pushed my bullying nature deep down into my unconscious mind because I did not want to admit that I, too, could be a bully. Other people had unconsciously mirrored exactly what I needed to see, because I had projected this capacity out onto them rather than seeing it within myself. They had, in fact, done me a favor; I just had not seen it at the time.

And maybe I had rarely bullied other people, but I had bullied myself pretty much all my life. I forced myself to do things I didn't want to do, eat things I didn't like, and say "nice" things at the expense of my inner knowing.

I knew I needed to get in contact with this side of myself. How was that going to happen when I was completely unaware of it?

The next day I went into meditative silence and asked my intuition to show me my inner bully. And he popped right up—a tall, venomous snake with a sharp tongue. He called himself "Billy the Bully."

Chagrined, I drew him in a sketch pad. He had bright, almost glowing yellow eyes.

Then I called a friend and talked for thirty minutes about my realization.

The next day I went back into meditative silence and asked for assistance with integrating this part of my personality so it would no longer attract other bullies to me. In my visualization, Billy the Bully was placed against my back, with his head arched over my head. I did not move; I allowed him to be there. Apparently, this needed to be done. After a period—I don't know how long—the snake dissolved into my spine and scalp. He became a part of me.

I knew his gifts included assertiveness, strength, and a brilliant eye for spotting what is not in integrity—qualities I now can better access.

PROMPTS TO GET YOU STARTED:

How can I better let others know what specific things I need from them?

Which of my relationships is the least supportive? What can I do about it, apart from playing the role of victim?

Who wears me out? How can I remedy that situation?

Do I do things for other people to please them or to control the situation in some way?

With whom do I need to set better boundaries to protect my well-being?

What conditioned responses to others leave me feeling less-than? What would be better responses for me to enact?

In what ways have I given my power away to others—through resignation, passivity, and depression? How can I stop that drain?

What unresolved relationships do I still have?

What family behavior patterns have I been repeating that might interfere with my body's ability to heal?

When I talk about my situation, do I focus on the illness or on how I am being helped?

What can I say "no" to, so I can say "yes" to what matters more to me?

How do I express my authentic self with members of my family? With my friends? How can I move toward greater authenticity in my interactions with them?

How willing am I to risk the disapproval of others to remain truthful to myself and my beliefs?

What activities would I like to do with family and friends?

How did I give love today?
How did I receive love today?

Which of my relationships bring me love, comfort, and peace?

Which of my relationships are the most supportive?

What can I do to ask for more support from others?

How can I improve my connections with others?

What do I still have to give to one or more persons?

How can I use cancer to widen my heart and increase my level of compassion for others?

If I could invite one person into a conversation with me, who would I choose, and what would I want to talk about?

Who do I care about most in the world, and what could I do today to make sure they know it?

If I were to write a letter to a loved one, what would I say?

Who do I know that reflects or symbolizes hope, resilience, courage, endurance, patience, fortitude, tenacity, heroism, strength? What does each quality look like? How can I better mirror each quality? Then how would my life look different?

How can I move toward feeling gratitude for exactly where I am right now in my cancer journey?

MOVING DEEPER:

There are three modes of operating in relationships that form a triangle: persecutor, martyr/victim, and rescuer. Martyrs might sacrifice themselves for their mates, their children, or their jobs, then become ill. Then they use the illness to persecute their mates into having to take care of them. Victims play helpless and believe they have no choices or choose not to make them. They fall into resignation and like to blame persecutors and look for rescuers, yet ironically resent it when others do assist them. Persecutors exact penance from victims and martyrs through veiled anger and guilt or resentment. It is easy to switch positions around the triangle with other significant people in our lives. Think back to a recent unhappy exchange with a loved one. Do I have a tendency to play the role of martyr, victim, rescuer, or persecutor in my own mind? What role did I play in the drama? How can I behave differently to avoid the triangular rupture? How can I avoid stepping into the triangle?

DIVE TO THRIVE:

What are my very deepest thoughts and feelings about a traumatic situation with a significant relationship? What happened? How did I feel about it then? How do I feel about it now? How did I change as a result of the pain? How did the event shape my character? Did it impact how I react in particular ways, and if so, how can I begin responding in more thoughtful ways instead? How can I find some peace with what occurred?

SOARING WITH SPIRIT

Two years after the sarcoma diagnosis and a third major surgery, I went to my post-operative appointment with a nurse practitioner. She said the tumor on the pulmonary vein next to my heart had grown from half an inch to 2.5 inches during the five weeks before that surgery.

"You need to get back on chemotherapy," she said.

I told her I had an orphan cancer and had run through all available chemotherapy agents known to benefit endometrial sarcoma patients.

She said she had seen situations like mine for thirty years. If there was no more chemo then I needed to get ready for Hospice.

I felt struck in the head.

(I later learned there was a clinical trial, but ironically I did not qualify for it because from that point forward I had no more evidence of the sarcoma.)

I needed to write about this. If the nurse was right, I would be in Hospice within a few months. Part of me could then relax and let everything go, even the books I wanted to write.

On the other hand, perhaps I had made enough recent changes in my life that I would become healthier.

Then fear and doubt crept in—I must be in deep denial to think any such thoughts.

Yet I had heard many stories of people with miraculous last-moment-type remissions. And many of the women I knew with similar cancers were living for years.

Perhaps I could live for years with occasional surgeries.

As I wrote, I began to gain some clarity around seeing possibilities. I had been doing everything I knew to do to extend my life. I asked for faith and trust, and to let go of fear and doubt. Something rose within me, a strength I had not suspected. If I was going to die, I was going to go out like a hero finally going home.

I surrendered to the illness, letting go of my attachment to the outcome of my situation. And ironically, the relentless sarcoma relinquished its hold. I have been free of evidence of sarcoma and free of treatment for it since 2011.

PROMPTS TO GET YOU STARTED:

How does the cancer impact my beliefs about the Divine?

How do I feel about the belief that it is the Divine who helps and heals?

How can I increase my love for the divine part within myself?

How would I feel if I viewed the cancer experience as a divine injury or as a profound invitation to wake up to my true Self? How would my life change as a result?

Just as the Divine is formless Spirit, so we inhabit bodies that are primarily composed of energy fields below the subatomic level that defy our macro-world understandings of form. Our souls, as well, cannot be seen in the world of objects. I believe they are intangible, timeless, and deathless. Because we are reflections of the Spirit, we are worthy of re-experiencing wholeness in our bodies and of receiving cures. If I were to compose a letter to my individual cancer cells, what would I write?

Affirmations are attempts at changing our core beliefs so we have better experiences of life. What would a good affirmation be for my situation?

Intentions involve decisions that help us move in particular directions. What are some of my intentions for myself?

What is a nighttime dream I have had recently? What might be its message for me?

Larry Dossey, MD, in his book *The Power of Prayer and the Practice of Medicine,* listed the characteristics that five Japanese cancer patients, who experienced spontaneous remissions, had in common. These characteristics included:

1. Having an existential crisis while living with cancer and choosing to resolve their crises themselves.

2. A surprising lack of anxiety and depression after their diagnoses. For four of the patients, this was connected with a strong religious faith.

3. Giving themselves completely to the will of the Divine and renewing their commitment to former activities and new interests. They intuited more meaning and a bigger picture in life's experiences, including the cancer.

4. Improving their relationships with others, which involved both personal growth and introspection.

5. A conspicuous spiritual viewpoint.

Write out this list. How do or don't I match up with each item? If there are any I don't match up with, what plan can I create to work on that item?

What am I willing to endure to be cured?

What does it mean to surrender to the Divine?

How much control do I really have over the process and results of my cancer journey?

MOVING DEEPER:

Write out a direct prayer to the Divine. Include a request and an expression of gratitude.

If I am experiencing a dark spiritual time, what pieces of myself that are deep within can I draw into the light to write about?

DIVE TO THRIVE:

What are my very deepest thoughts and feelings about an extremely important spiritual issue that has affected me and my life? Was I pushed into a certain set of religious beliefs or behaviors that did not fit my authentic self? How did I feel about it then? How do I feel about it now? How did the event shape my character? Did it impact how I react in particular ways, and if so, how can I begin responding in more thoughtful ways instead? How can I find some peace with what occurred?

Source:

1. Dossey, Larry. *Healing Words: The Power of Prayer and the Practice of Medicine.* San Francisco: Harper San Francisco, 1993:241-242.

4

FINAL DIVE TO THRIVE

O O

In *The Power Principle: Influence with Honor,* author Blaine Lee explains that we have integrity when our thoughts, feelings, words, and actions are aligned and cohesive. In what ways can I bring greater alignment among these aspects of myself?

What parts of myself have I lost along the road of life? How can I regain them?

What is the worst thing that ever happened to me? How did I feel about it then? How do I feel about it now? What healing options do I have available to me? How did the event shape my character? Did it impact how I react in particular ways, and if so, how can I begin responding in more thoughtful ways instead? How can I find some peace with what occurred?

MY GREAT HOPE

My great hope is that, with the guidance of a mental health professional, you are able to use these prompts as springboards to find resources, knowledge, and wisdom within yourself. May these give rise to healing, greater equanimity, and possibly even a shedding of the disease.

Source:

1. Lee, Blaine. *The Power Principle: Influence with Honor* (New York: Simon & Schuster, May 15, 1997) Page 166.

www.ingramcontent.com/pod-product-compliance
Lightning Source LLC
Chambersburg PA
CBHW011536260326
41914CB00008B/1175